My Pregnancy Journal

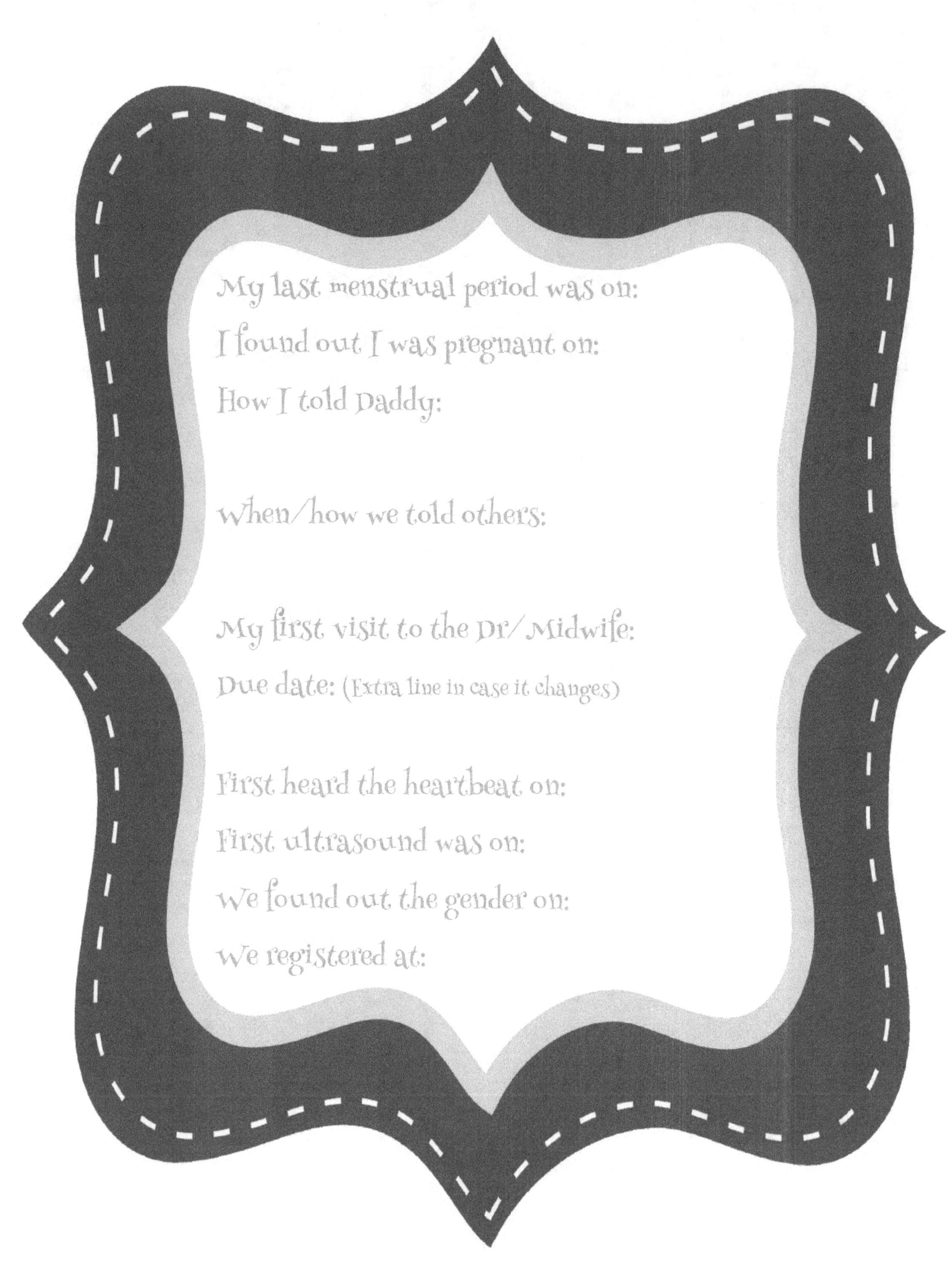

My last menstrual period was on:
I found out I was pregnant on:
How I told Daddy:

When/how we told others:

My first visit to the Dr/Midwife:
Due date: (Extra line in case it changes)

First heard the heartbeat on:
First ultrasound was on:
We found out the gender on:
We registered at:

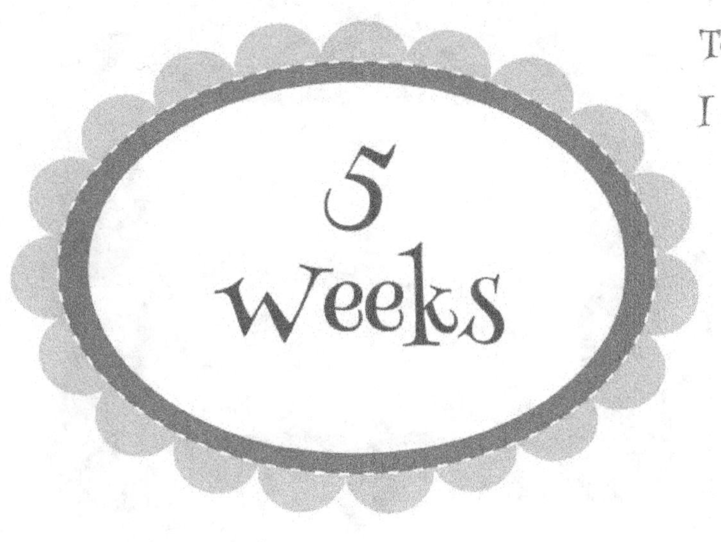

Today's Date:

I am feeling:

Baby is the size of a:

Showing:

I have (circle) lost/gained _______ lbs and my belly measures:

Gender:

I am craving:

Maternity clothes:

My emotions are:

I can't stand the sight of:

I can't wait to:

We like the names:

My sleep patterns are:

Movement:

I miss:

My skin is:

I'm reading, watching, listening, etc.:

This week baby is growing so fast! He or she began:

This week we had the memory of:

Today's Date:

I am feeling:

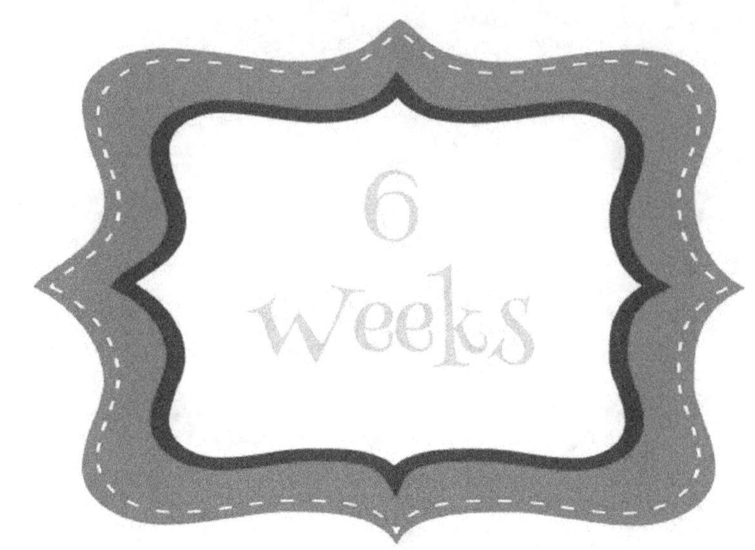

Baby is the size of a:

Showing:

I have (circle) lost/gained ______ lbs and my belly measures:

Gender:

I am craving:

Maternity clothes:

My emotions are:

I can't stand the sight of:

I can't wait to:

We like the names:

My sleep patterns are:

Movement:

I miss:

My skin is:

I'm reading, watching, listening, etc.:

This week baby is growing so fast! He or she began:

This week we had the memory of:

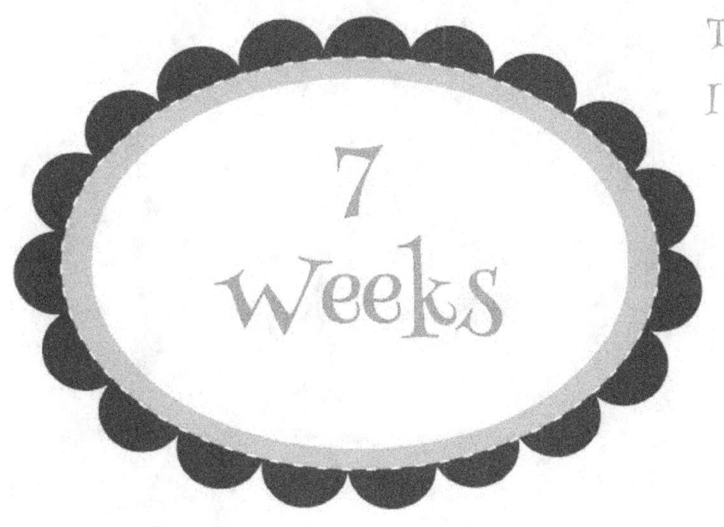

Today's Date:

I am feeling:

Baby is the size of a:

Showing:

I have (circle) lost/gained ______ lbs and my belly measures:

Gender:

I am craving:

Maternity clothes:

My emotions are:

I can't stand the sight of:

I can't wait to:

We like the names:

My sleep patterns are:

Movement:

I miss:

My skin is:

I'm reading, watching, listening, etc.:

This week baby is growing so fast! He or she began:

This week we had the memory of:

Today's Date:
I am feeling:

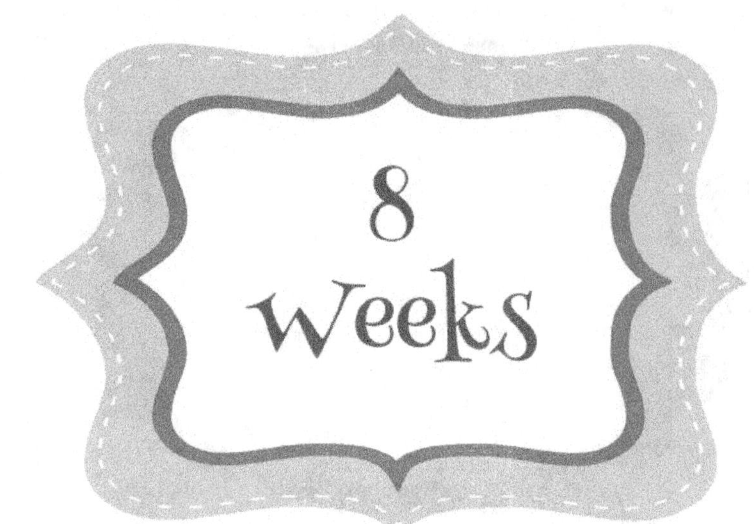

Baby is the size of a:
Showing:
I have (circle) lost/gained _______ lbs and my belly measures:
Gender:
I am craving:

Maternity clothes:
My emotions are:
I can't stand the sight of:
I can't wait to:
We like the names:
My sleep patterns are:
Movement:
I miss:
My skin is:
I'm reading, watching, listening, etc.:
This week baby is growing so fast! He or she began:

This week we had the memory of:

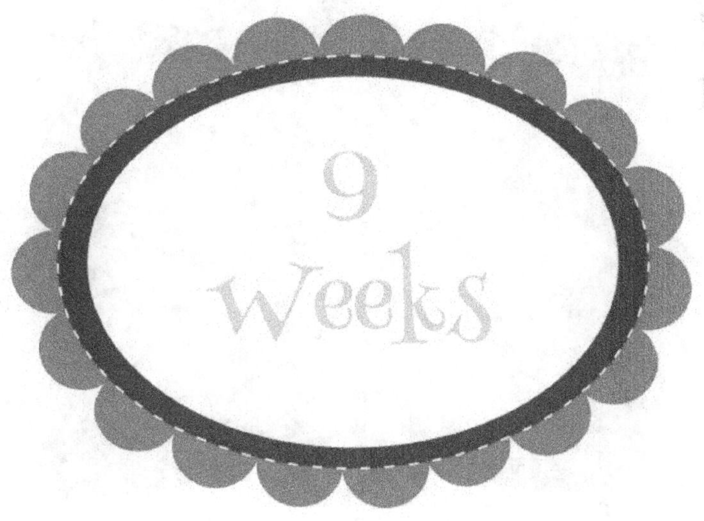

Baby is the size of a:

Showing:

I have (circle) lost / gained ______ lbs and my belly measures:

Gender:

I am craving:

Maternity clothes:

My emotions are:

I can't stand the sight of:

I can't wait to:

We like the names:

My sleep patterns are:

Movement:

I miss:

My skin is:

I'm reading, watching, listening, etc.:

This week baby is growing so fast! He or she began:

This week we had the memory of:

Today's Date:

I am feeling:

Baby is the size of a:

Showing:

I have (circle) lost/gained ________ lbs and my belly measures:

Gender:

I am craving:

Maternity clothes:

My emotions are:

I can't stand the sight of:

I can't wait to:

We like the names:

My sleep patterns are:

Movement:

I miss:

My skin is:

I'm reading, watching, listening, etc.:

This week baby is growing so fast! He or she began:

This week we had the memory of:

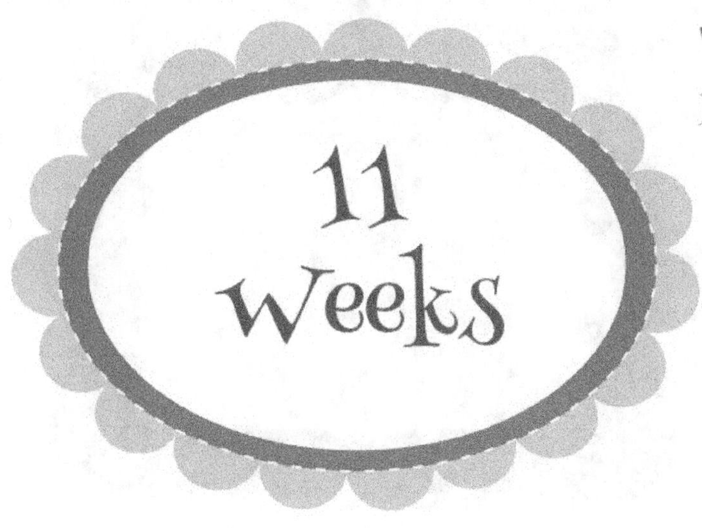

Today's Date:

I am feeling:

Baby is the size of a:

Showing:

I have (circle) lost/gained _______ lbs and my belly measures:

Gender:

I am craving:

Maternity clothes:

My emotions are:

I can't stand the sight of:

I can't wait to:

We like the names:

My sleep patterns are:

Movement:

I miss:

My skin is:

I'm reading, watching, listening, etc.:

This week baby is growing so fast! He or she began:

This week we had the memory of:

Today's Date:

I am feeling:

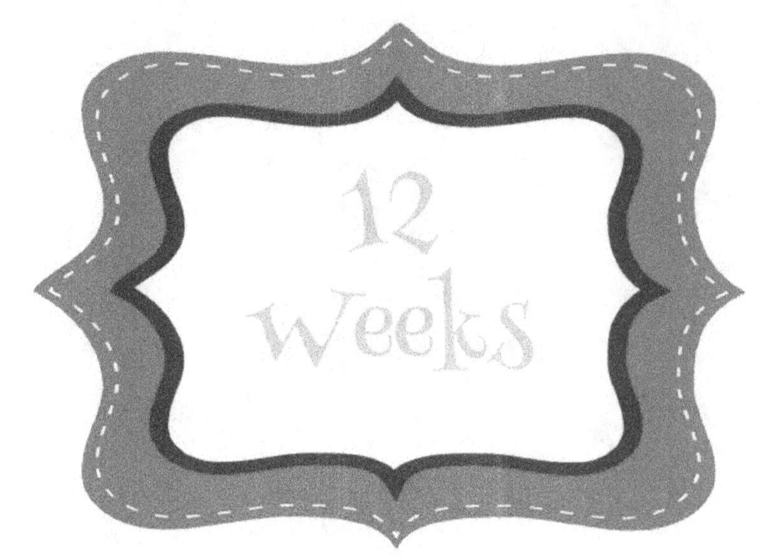

Baby is the size of a:

Showing:

I have (circle) lost/gained _______ lbs and my belly measures:

Gender:

I am craving:

Maternity clothes:

My emotions are:

I can't stand the sight of:

I can't wait to:

We like the names:

My sleep patterns are:

Movement:

I miss:

My skin is:

I'm reading, watching, listening, etc.:

This week baby is growing so fast! He or she began:

This week we had the memory of:

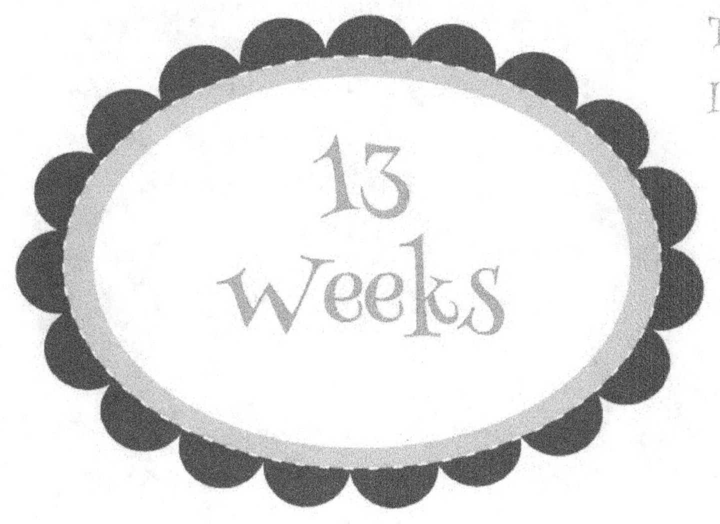

Today's Date:

I am feeling:

Baby is the size of a:

Showing:

I have (circle) lost/gained _______ lbs and my belly measures:

Gender:

I am craving:

Maternity clothes:

My emotions are:

I can't stand the sight of:

I can't wait to:

We like the names:

My sleep patterns are:

Movement:

I miss:

My skin is:

I'm reading, watching, listening, etc.:

This week baby is growing so fast! He or she began:

This week we had the memory of:

Today's Date:

I am feeling:

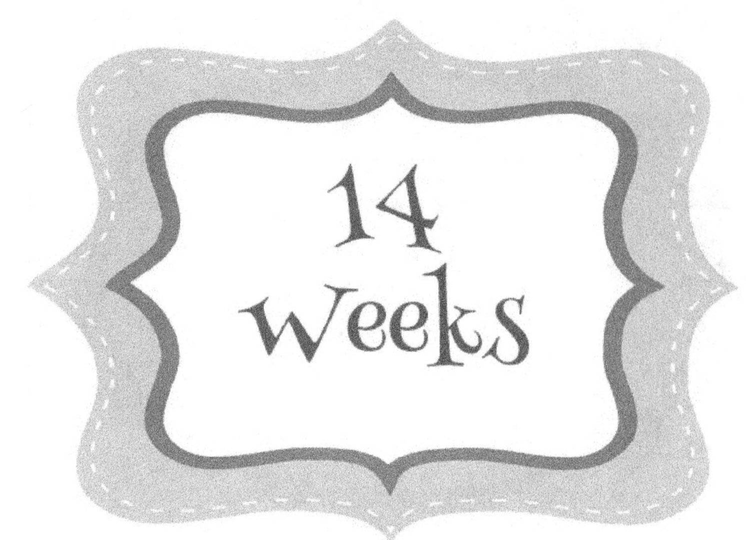

Baby is the size of a:

Showing:

I have (circle) lost/gained _______ lbs and my belly measures:

Gender:

I am craving:

Maternity clothes:

My emotions are:

I can't stand the sight of:

I can't wait to:

We like the names:

My sleep patterns are:

Movement:

I miss:

My skin is:

I'm reading, watching, listening, etc.:

This week baby is growing so fast! He or she began:

This week we had the memory of:

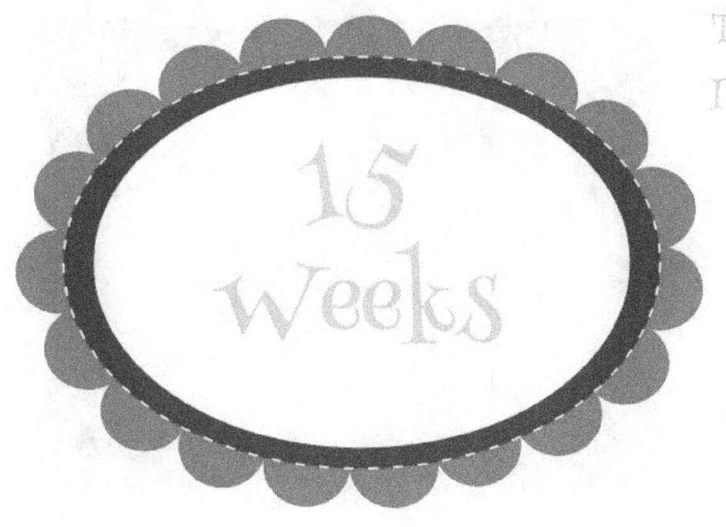

Today's Date:

I am feeling:

Baby is the size of a:

Showing:

I have (circle) lost/gained _______ lbs and my belly measures:

Gender:

I am craving:

Maternity clothes:

My emotions are:

I can't stand the sight of:

I can't wait to:

We like the names:

My sleep patterns are:

Movement:

I miss:

My skin is:

I'm reading, watching, listening, etc.:

This week baby is growing so fast! He or she began:

This week we had the memory of:

Today's Date:

I am feeling:

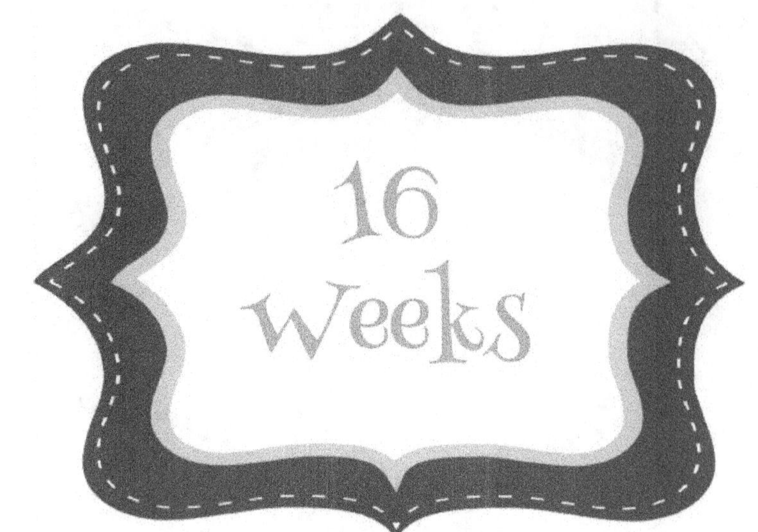

Baby is the size of a:

Showing:

I have (circle) lost/gained _______ lbs and my belly measures:

Gender:

I am craving:

Maternity clothes:

My emotions are:

I can't stand the sight of:

I can't wait to:

We like the names:

My sleep patterns are:

Movement:

I miss:

My skin is:

I'm reading, watching, listening, etc.:

This week baby is growing so fast! He or she began:

This week we had the memory of:

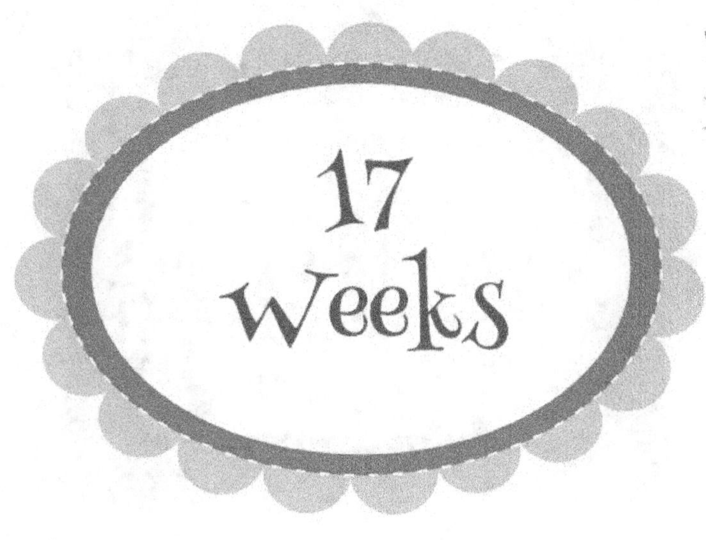

Today's Date:

I am feeling:

Baby is the size of a:

Showing:

I have (circle) lost/gained _______ lbs and my belly measures:

Gender:

I am craving:

Maternity clothes:

My emotions are:

I can't stand the sight of:

I can't wait to:

We like the names:

My sleep patterns are:

Movement:

I miss:

My skin is:

I'm reading, watching, listening, etc.:

This week baby is growing so fast! He or she began:

This week we had the memory of:

Today's Date:
I am feeling:

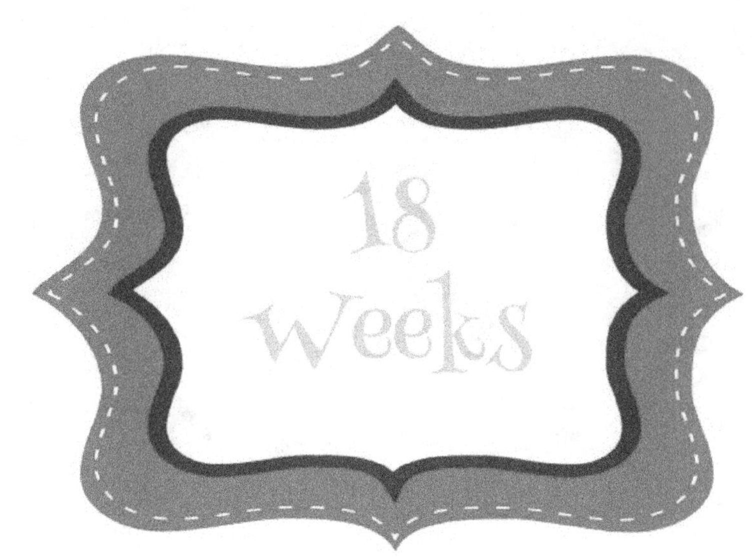

Baby is the size of a:
Showing:
I have (circle) lost/gained _______ lbs and my belly measures:
Gender:
I am craving:

Maternity clothes:
My emotions are:
I can't stand the sight of:
I can't wait to:
We like the names:
My sleep patterns are:
Movement:
I miss:
My skin is:
I'm reading, watching, listening, etc.:
This week baby is growing so fast! He or she began:

This week we had the memory of:

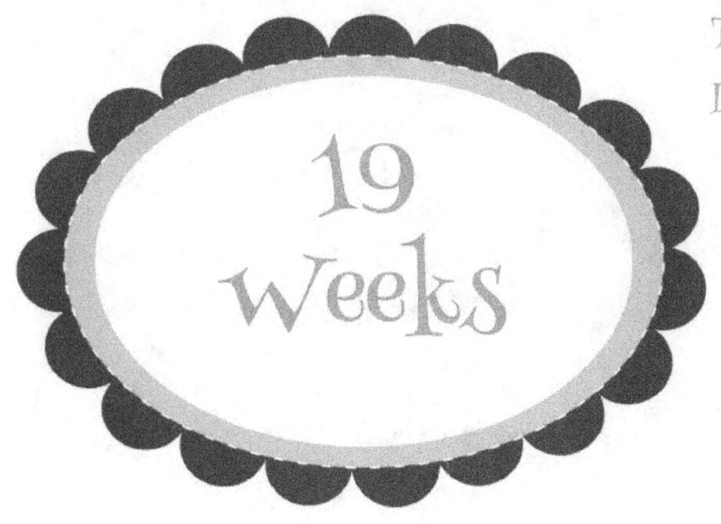

Today's Date:

I am feeling:

Baby is the size of a:

Showing:

I have (circle) lost/gained _______ lbs and my belly measures:

Gender:

I am craving:

Maternity clothes:

My emotions are:

I can't stand the sight of:

I can't wait to:

We like the names:

My sleep patterns are:

Movement:

I miss:

My skin is:

I'm reading, watching, listening, etc.:

This week baby is growing so fast! He or she began:

This week we had the memory of:

Today's Date:

I am feeling:

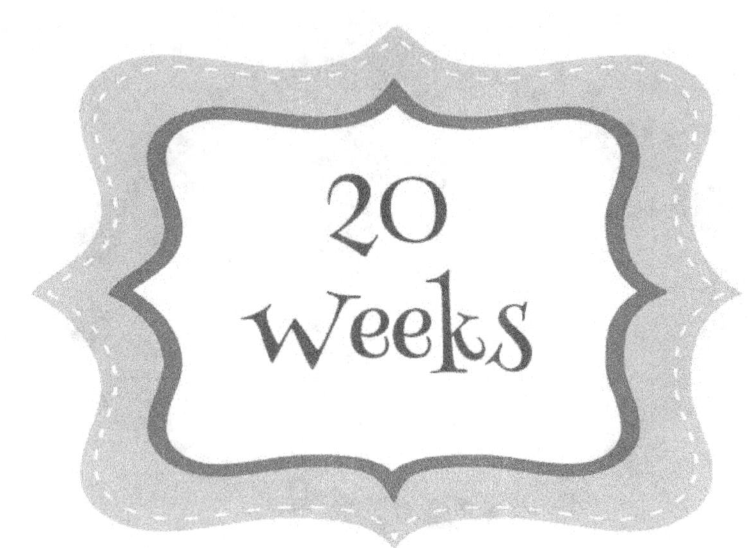

Baby is the size of a:

Showing:

I have (circle) lost/gained _______lbs and my belly measures:

Gender:

I am craving:

Maternity clothes:

My emotions are:

I can't stand the sight of:

I can't wait to:

We like the names:

My sleep patterns are:

Movement:

I miss:

My skin is:

I'm reading, watching, listening, etc.:

This week baby is growing so fast! He or she began:

This week we had the memory of:

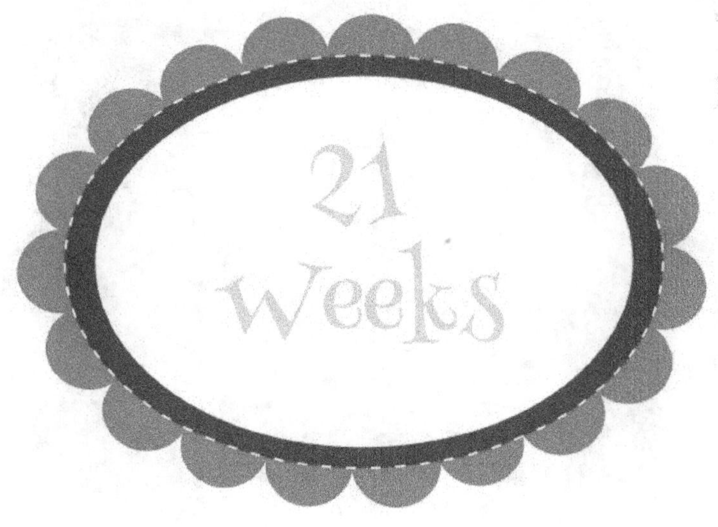

Today's Date:

I am feeling:

Baby is the size of a:

Showing:

I have (circle) lost/gained _______ lbs and my belly measures:

Gender:

I am craving:

Maternity clothes:

My emotions are:

I can't stand the sight of:

I can't wait to:

We like the names:

My sleep patterns are:

Movement:

I miss:

My skin is:

I'm reading, watching, listening, etc.:

This week baby is growing so fast! He or she began:

This week we had the memory of:

Today's Date:

I am feeling:

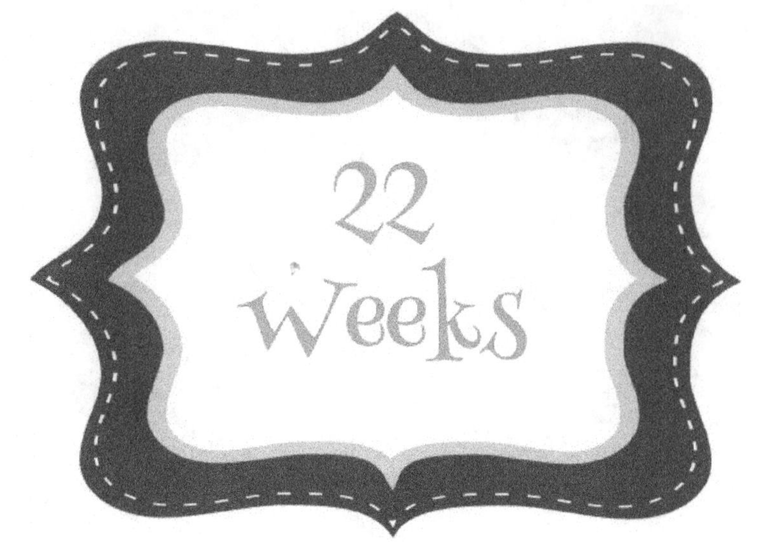

Baby is the size of a:

Showing:

I have (circle) lost/gained _______ lbs and my belly measures:

Gender:

I am craving:

Maternity clothes:

My emotions are:

I can't stand the sight of:

I can't wait to:

We like the names:

My sleep patterns are:

Movement:

I miss:

My skin is:

I'm reading, watching, listening, etc.:

This week baby is growing so fast! He or she began:

This week we had the memory of:

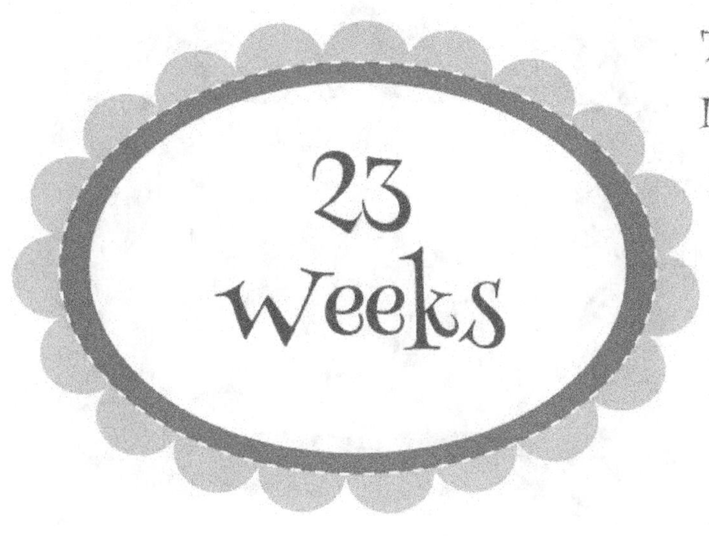

Today's Date:

I am feeling:

Baby is the size of a:

Showing:

I have (circle) lost/gained _______ lbs and my belly measures:

Gender:

I am craving:

Maternity clothes:

My emotions are:

I can't stand the sight of:

I can't wait to:

We like the names:

My sleep patterns are:

Movement:

I miss:

My skin is:

I'm reading, watching, listening, etc.:

This week baby is growing so fast! He or she began:

This week we had the memory of:

Today's Date:

I am feeling:

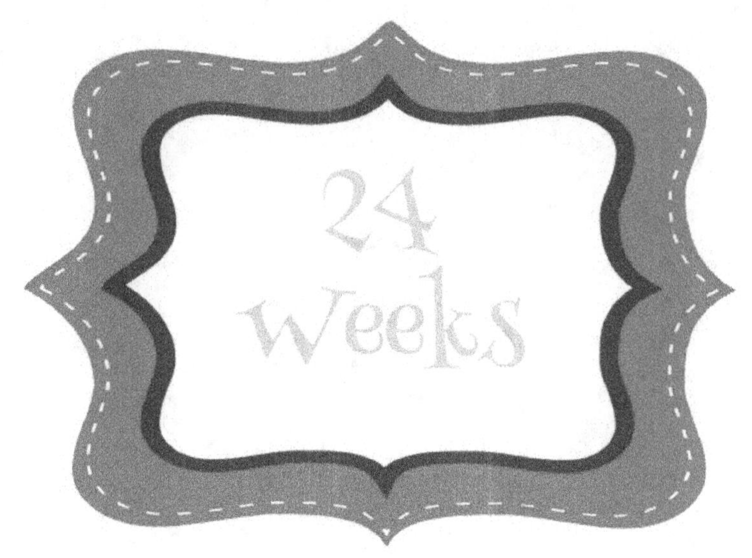

Baby is the size of a:

Showing:

I have (circle) lost/gained ________ lbs and my belly measures:

Gender:

I am craving:

Maternity clothes:

My emotions are:

I can't stand the sight of:

I can't wait to:

We like the names:

My sleep patterns are:

Movement:

I miss:

My skin is:

I'm reading, watching, listening, etc.:

This week baby is growing so fast! He or she began:

This week we had the memory of:

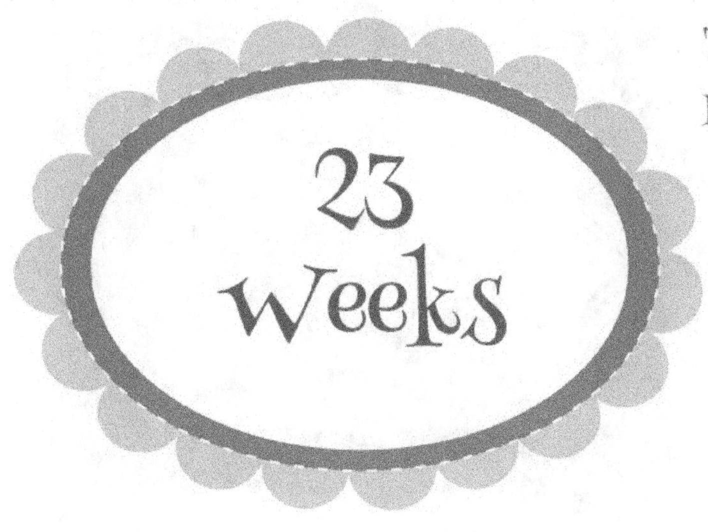

Today's Date:

I am feeling:

Baby is the size of a:

Showing:

I have (circle) lost/gained _______ lbs and my belly measures:

Gender:

I am craving:

Maternity clothes:

My emotions are:

I can't stand the sight of:

I can't wait to:

We like the names:

My sleep patterns are:

Movement:

I miss:

My skin is:

I'm reading, watching, listening, etc.:

This week baby is growing so fast! He or she began:

This week we had the memory of:

Today's Date:

I am feeling:

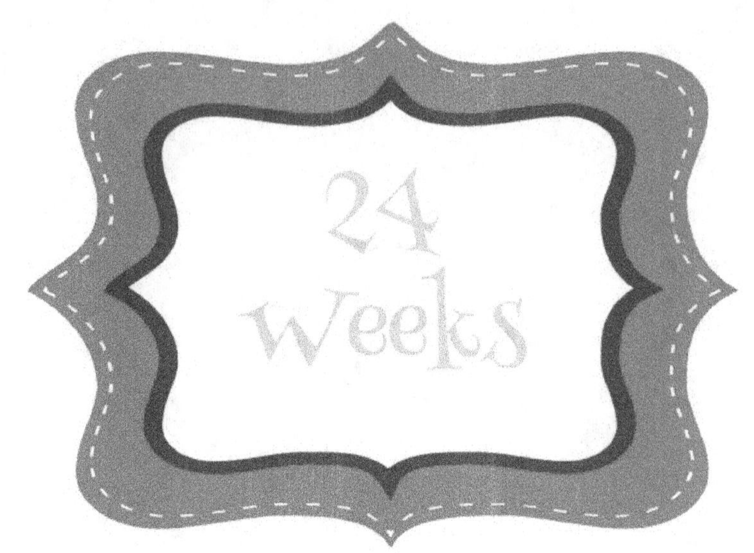

Baby is the size of a:

Showing:

I have (circle) lost/gained _______ lbs and my belly measures:

Gender:

I am craving:

Maternity clothes:

My emotions are:

I can't stand the sight of:

I can't wait to:

We like the names:

My sleep patterns are:

Movement:

I miss:

My skin is:

I'm reading, watching, listening, etc.:

This week baby is growing so fast! He or she began:

This week we had the memory of:

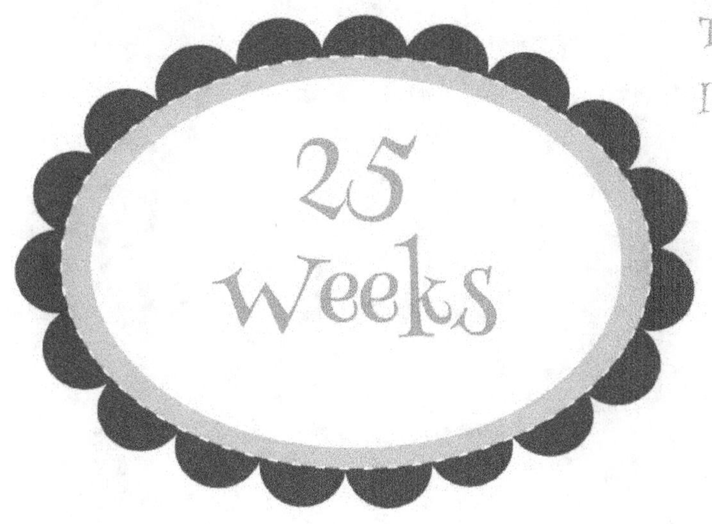

Today's Date:

I am feeling:

Baby is the size of a:

Showing:

I have (circle) lost/gained _______ lbs and my belly measures:

Gender:

I am craving:

Maternity clothes:

My emotions are:

I can't stand the sight of:

I can't wait to:

We like the names:

My sleep patterns are:

Movement:

I miss:

My skin is:

I'm reading, watching, listening, etc.:

This week baby is growing so fast! He or she began:

This week we had the memory of:

Today's Date:

I am feeling:

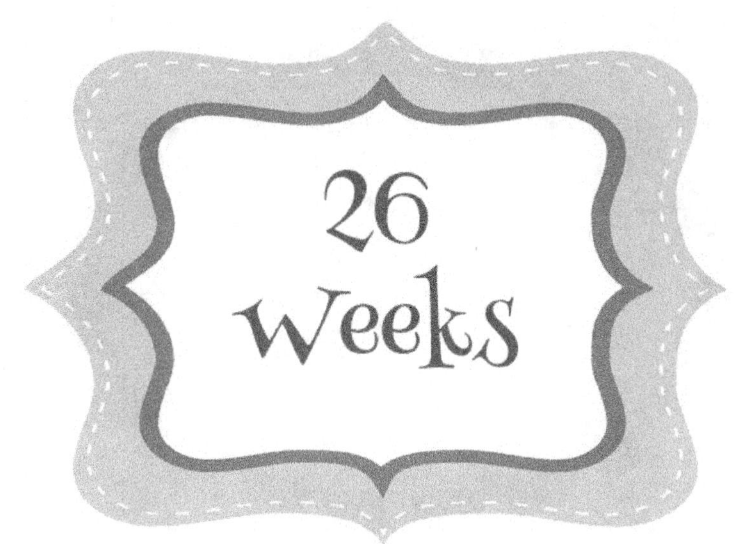

Baby is the size of a:

Showing:

I have (circle) lost/gained _______lbs and my belly measures:

Gender:

I am craving:

Maternity clothes:

My emotions are:

I can't stand the sight of:

I can't wait to:

We like the names:

My sleep patterns are:

Movement:

I miss:

My skin is:

I'm reading, watching, listening, etc.:

This week baby is growing so fast! He or she began:

This week we had the memory of:

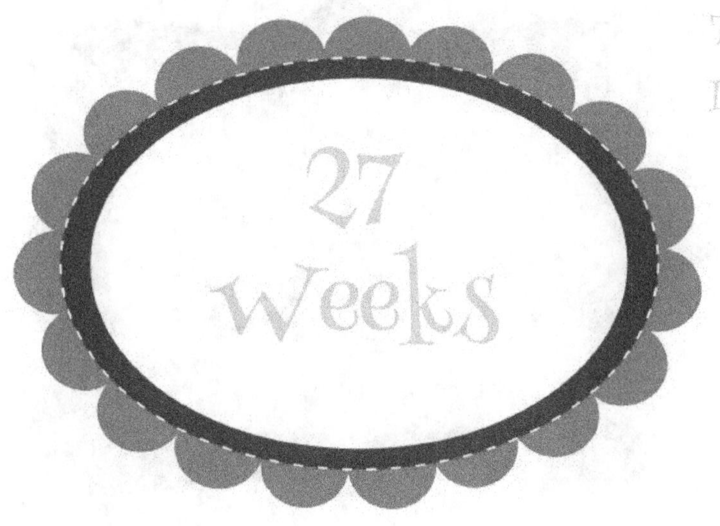

Today's Date:

I am feeling:

Baby is the size of a:

Showing:

I have (circle) lost / gained _______ lbs and my belly measures:

Gender:

I am craving:

Maternity clothes:

My emotions are:

I can't stand the sight of:

I can't wait to:

We like the names:

My sleep patterns are:

Movement:

I miss:

My skin is:

I'm reading, watching, listening, etc.:

This week baby is growing so fast! He or she began:

This week we had the memory of:

Today's Date:

I am feeling:

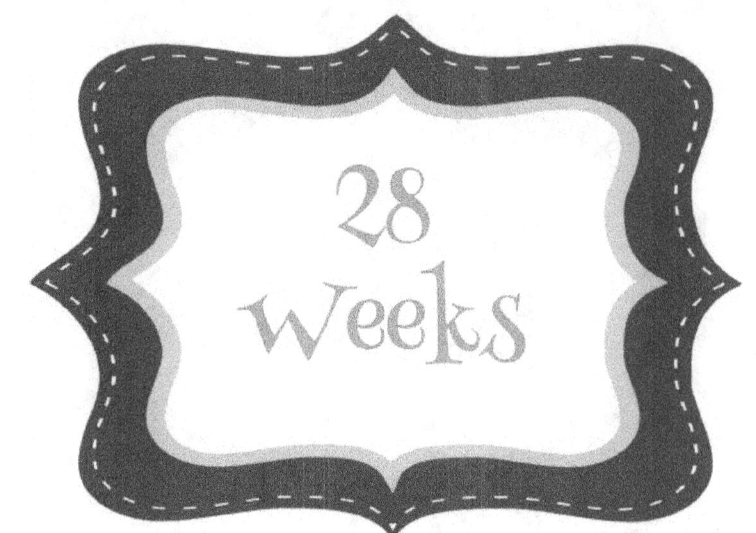

Baby is the size of a:

Showing:

I have (circle) lost/gained _______ lbs and my belly measures:

Gender:

I am craving:

Maternity clothes:

My emotions are:

I can't stand the sight of:

I can't wait to:

We like the names:

My sleep patterns are:

Movement:

I miss:

My skin is:

I'm reading, watching, listening, etc.:

This week baby is growing so fast! He or she began:

This week we had the memory of:

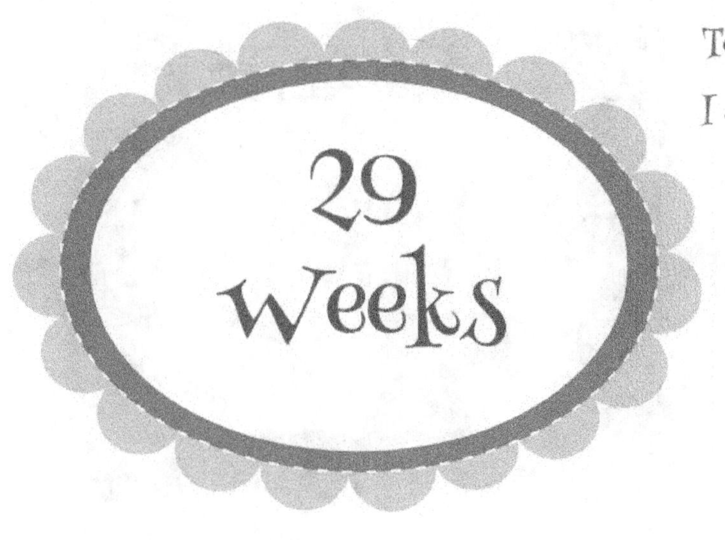

Today's Date:

I am feeling:

Baby is the size of a:

Showing:

I have (circle) lost/gained ______ lbs and my belly measures:

Gender:

I am craving:

Maternity clothes:

My emotions are:

I can't stand the sight of:

I can't wait to:

We like the names:

My sleep patterns are:

Movement:

I miss:

My skin is:

I'm reading, watching, listening, etc.:

This week baby is growing so fast! He or she began:

This week we had the memory of:

Today's Date:

I am feeling:

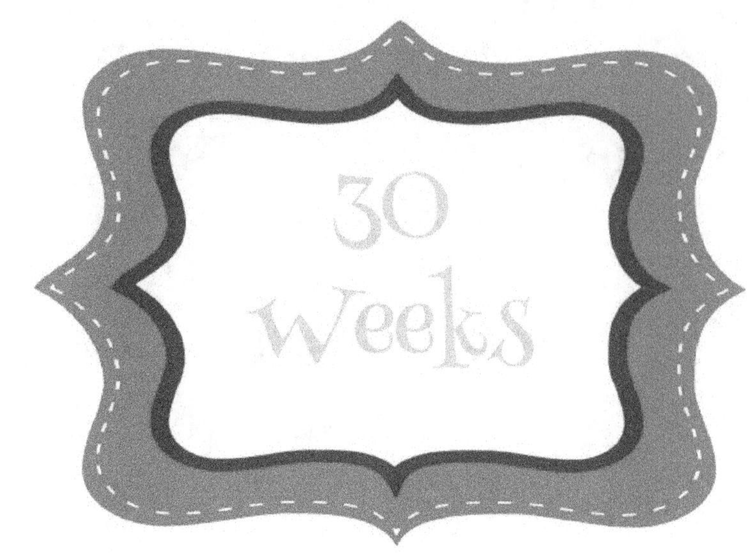

Baby is the size of a:

Showing:

I have (circle) lost/gained _______ lbs and my belly measures:

Gender:

I am craving:

Maternity clothes:

My emotions are:

I can't stand the sight of:

I can't wait to:

We like the names:

My sleep patterns are:

Movement:

I miss:

My skin is:

I'm reading, watching, listening, etc.:

This week baby is growing so fast! He or she began:

This week we had the memory of:

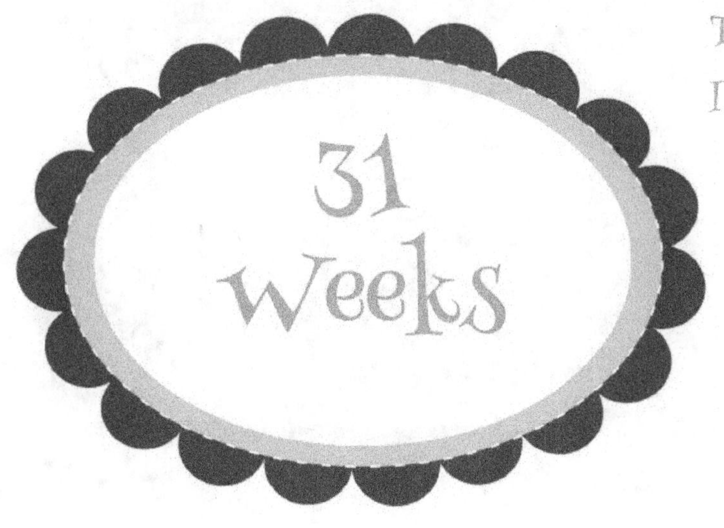

Today's Date:

I am feeling:

Baby is the size of a:

Showing:

I have (circle) lost/gained _______ lbs and my belly measures:

Gender:

I am craving:

Maternity clothes:

My emotions are:

I can't stand the sight of:

I can't wait to:

We like the names:

My sleep patterns are:

Movement:

I miss:

My skin is:

I'm reading, watching, listening, etc.:

This week baby is growing so fast! He or she began:

This week we had the memory of:

Today's Date:

I am feeling:

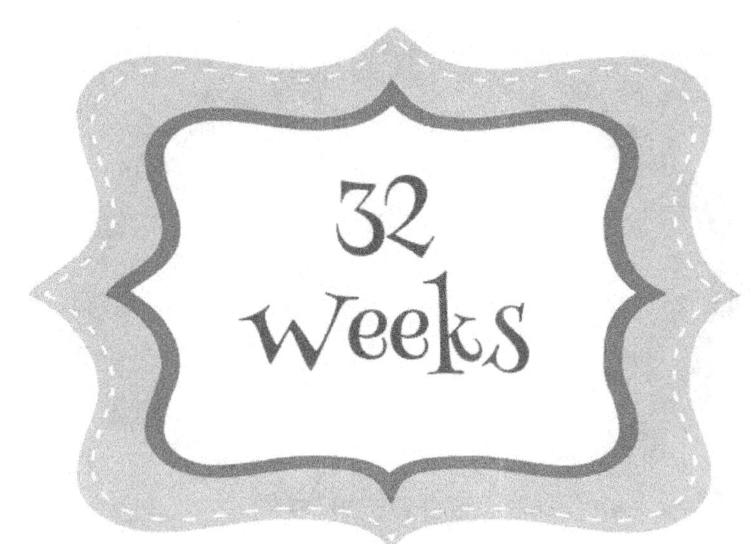

Baby is the size of a:

Showing:

I have (circle) lost/gained _______ lbs and my belly measures:

Gender:

I am craving:

Maternity clothes:

My emotions are:

I can't stand the sight of:

I can't wait to:

We like the names:

My sleep patterns are:

Movement:

I miss:

My skin is:

I'm reading, watching, listening, etc.:

This week baby is growing so fast! He or she began:

This week we had the memory of:

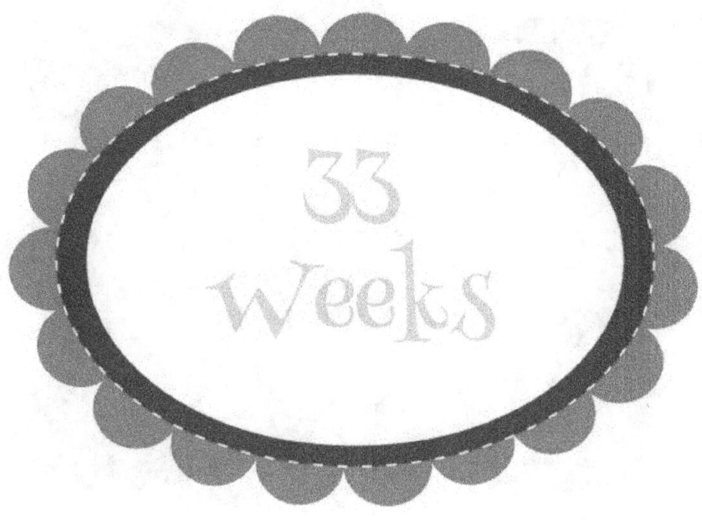

Today's Date:

I am feeling:

Baby is the size of a:

Showing:

I have (circle) lost/gained _______ lbs and my belly measures:

Gender:

I am craving:

Maternity clothes:

My emotions are:

I can't stand the sight of:

I can't wait to:

We like the names:

My sleep patterns are:

Movement:

I miss:

My skin is:

I'm reading, watching, listening, etc.:

This week baby is growing so fast! He or she began:

This week we had the memory of:

Today's Date:

I am feeling:

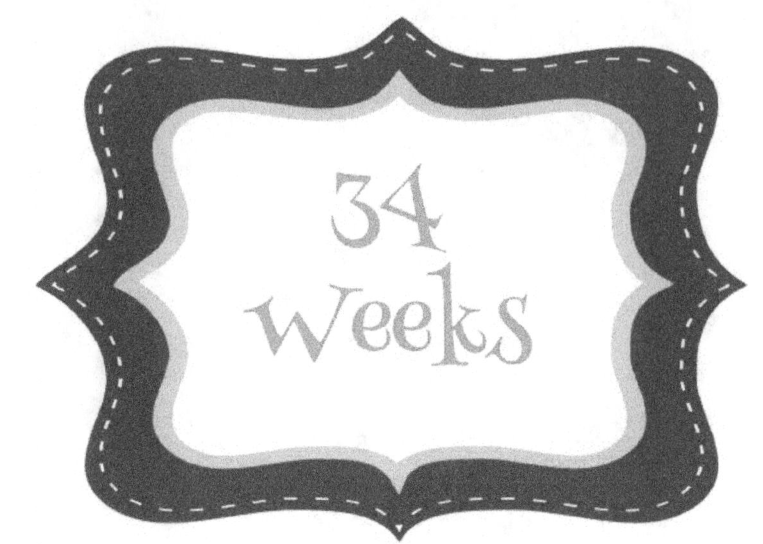

Baby is the size of a:

Showing:

I have (circle) lost/gained _______ lbs and my belly measures:

Gender:

I am craving:

Maternity clothes:

My emotions are:

I can't stand the sight of:

I can't wait to:

We like the names:

My sleep patterns are:

Movement:

I miss:

My skin is:

I'm reading, watching, listening, etc.:

This week baby is growing so fast! He or she began:

This week we had the memory of:

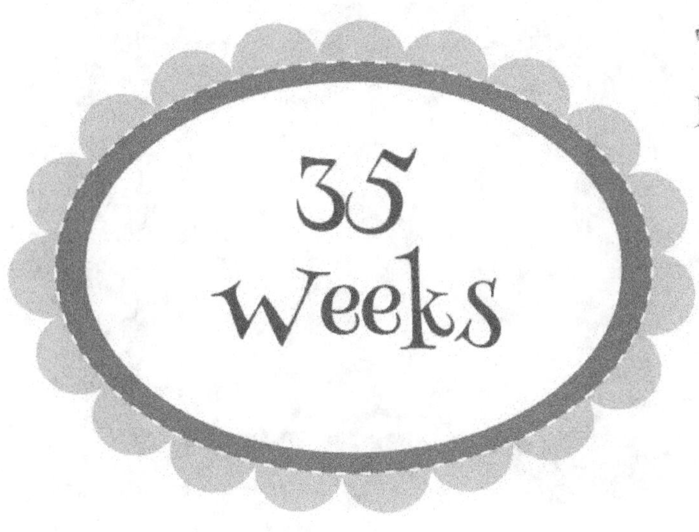

Today's Date:

I am feeling:

Baby is the size of a:

Showing:

I have (circle) lost/gained _______ lbs and my belly measures:

Gender:

I am craving:

Maternity clothes:

My emotions are:

I can't stand the sight of:

I can't wait to:

We like the names:

My sleep patterns are:

Movement:

I miss:

My skin is:

I'm reading, watching, listening, etc.:

This week baby is growing so fast! He or she began:

This week we had the memory of:

Today's Date:

I am feeling:

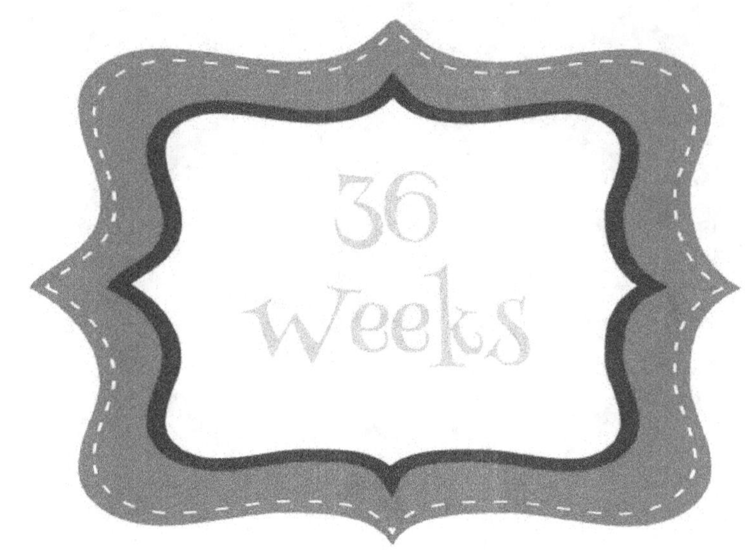

Baby is the size of a:

Showing:

I have (circle) lost/gained _______ lbs and my belly measures:

Gender:

I am craving:

Maternity clothes:

My emotions are:

I can't stand the sight of:

I can't wait to:

We like the names:

My sleep patterns are:

Movement:

I miss:

My skin is:

I'm reading, watching, listening, etc.:

This week baby is growing so fast! He or she began:

This week we had the memory of:

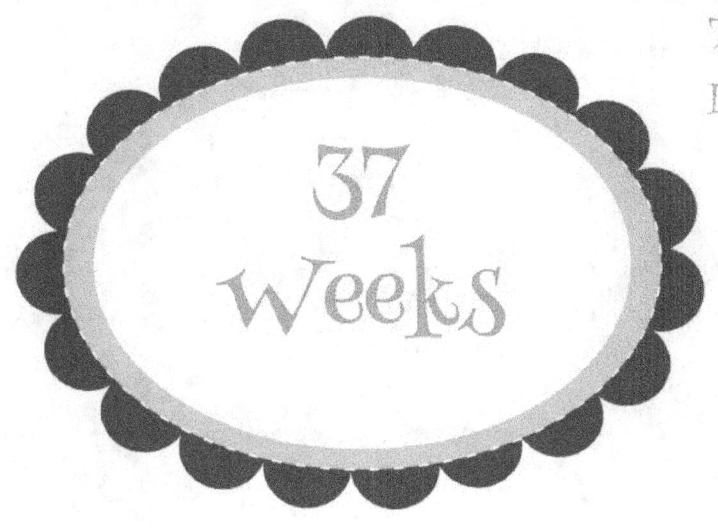

Today's Date:

I am feeling:

Baby is the size of a:

Showing:

I have (circle) lost/gained _______ lbs and my belly measures:

Gender:

I am craving:

Maternity clothes:

My emotions are:

I can't stand the sight of:

I can't wait to:

We like the names:

My sleep patterns are:

Movement:

I miss:

My skin is:

I'm reading, watching, listening, etc.:

This week baby is growing so fast! He or she began:

This week we had the memory of:

Today's Date:

I am feeling:

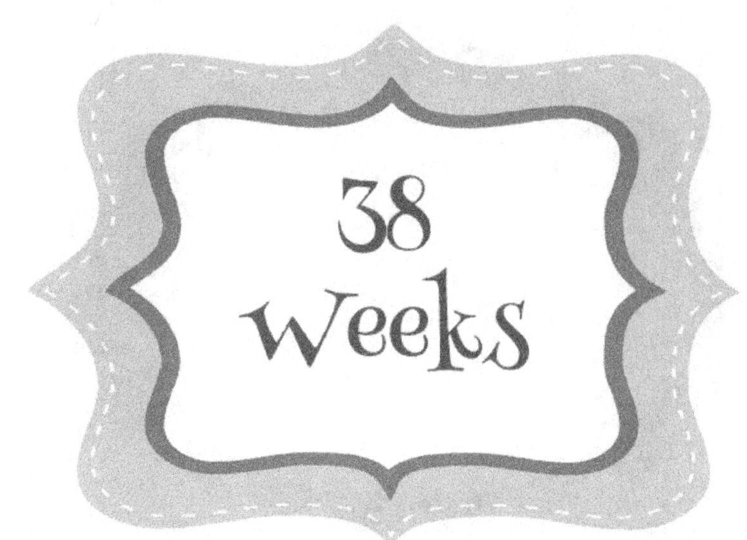

Baby is the size of a:

Showing:

I have (circle) lost/gained _______ lbs and my belly measures:

Gender:

I am craving:

Maternity clothes:

My emotions are:

I can't stand the sight of:

I can't wait to:

We like the names:

My sleep patterns are:

Movement:

I miss:

My skin is:

I'm reading, watching, listening, etc.:

This week baby is growing so fast! He or she began:

This week we had the memory of:

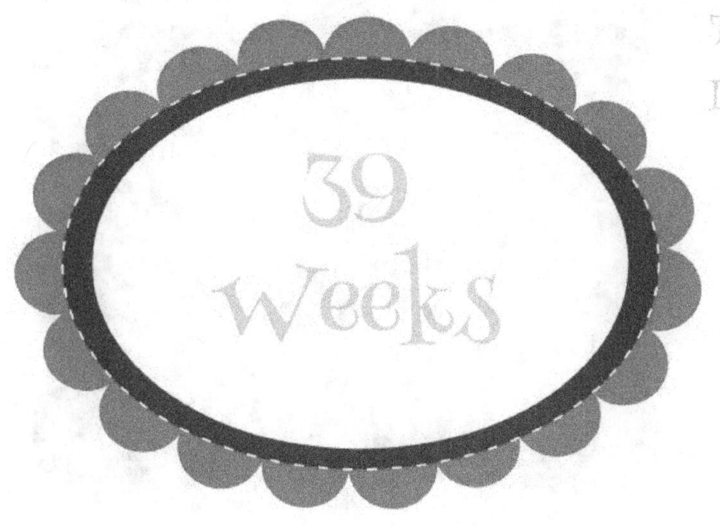

Today's Date:

I am feeling:

Baby is the size of a:

Showing:

I have (circle) lost/gained _______ lbs and my belly measures:

Gender:

I am craving:

Maternity clothes:

My emotions are:

I can't stand the sight of:

I can't wait to:

We like the names:

My sleep patterns are:

Movement:

I miss:

My skin is:

I'm reading, watching, listening, etc.:

This week baby is growing so fast! He or she began:

This week we had the memory of:

Today's Date:

I am feeling:

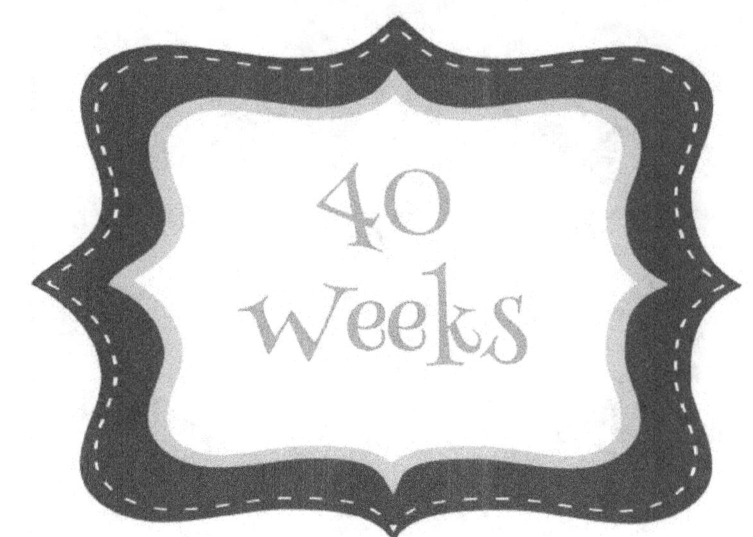

Baby is the size of a:

Showing:

I have (circle) lost/gained _______ lbs and my belly measures:

Gender:

I am craving:

Maternity clothes:

My emotions are:

I can't stand the sight of:

I can't wait to:

We like the names:

My sleep patterns are:

Movement:

I miss:

My skin is:

I'm reading, watching, listening, etc.:

This week baby is growing so fast! He or she began:

This week we had the memory of:

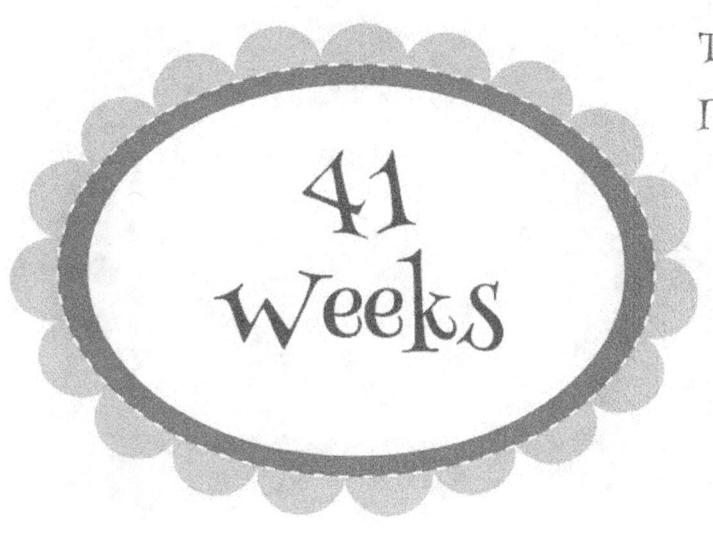

Today's Date:

I am feeling:

Baby is the size of a:

Showing:

I have (circle) lost/gained _______ lbs and my belly measures:

Gender:

I am craving:

Maternity clothes:

My emotions are:

I can't stand the sight of:

I can't wait to:

We like the names:

My sleep patterns are:

Movement:

I miss:

My skin is:

I'm reading, watching, listening, etc.:

This week baby is growing so fast! He or she began:

This week we had the memory of:

Today's Date:

I am feeling:

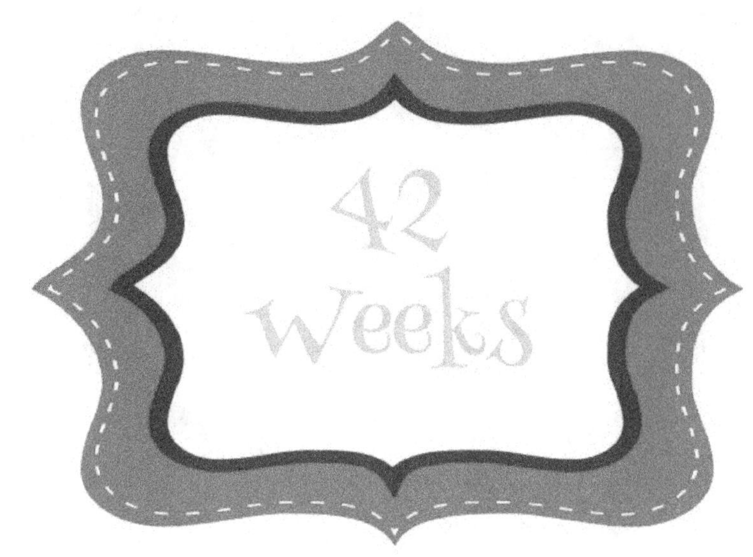

Baby is the size of a:

Showing:

I have (circle) lost/gained ________ lbs and my belly measures:

Gender:

I am craving:

Maternity clothes:

My emotions are:

I can't stand the sight of:

I can't wait to:

We like the names:

My sleep patterns are:

Movement:

I miss:

My skin is:

I'm reading, watching, listening, etc.:

This week baby is growing so fast! He or she began:

This week we had the memory of:

www.ingramcontent.com/pod-product-compliance
Lightning Source LLC
Chambersburg PA
CBHW081323250726
48662CB00008B/2726